FAITH, HOPE AND LUCK

A Sociological Study of Children Growing Up with a Life-Threatening Illness

Charles Waddell

UNIVERSITY
PRESS OF
AMERICA

Copyright © 1983 by

University Press of America, Inc.™

P.O. Box 19101, Washington, D.C. 20036

Printed in the United States of America

Library of Congress Cataloging in Publication Data

Waddell, Charles.
    Faith, hope, and luck, a sociological study of
children growing up with a life-threatening illness.

    Bibliography: p.
    1. Cystic fibrosis--Social aspects. 2. Cystic
fibrosis--Psychological aspects. 3. Terminally ill
children--Psychology. 4. Chronic diseases in children--
Social aspects. 5. Chronic diseases in children--
Psychological aspects. I. Title.
RJ456.C9W3   1983   305'.90814   82-24871
ISBN 0-8191-3011-7
ISBN 0-8191-3012-5 (pbk.)

FOR VIVIENNE AND GREGORY

ACKNOWLEDGEMENTS

Chapter Three originally appeared in slightly different form in *The Sociology of Health and Illness*, 4, 2 (July, 1982). It is reprinted here with the permission of the publisher, Routledge and Kegan Paul Ltd., London.

I wish to acknowledge the many helpful comments and criticisms I have had on this monograph from my colleagues Professors R. M. Berndt and B. L. Sansom and Dr. J. L. Gordon of the Department of Anthropology, University of Western Australia. I also thank Professors L. Broom, G. Vernon, Drs. R. Hill, J. Krol, K. Palmer, Ms. V. Florence and Ms. C. Warren for their suggestions on parts of the manuscript. Finally, my thanks to Vivienne, my wife, for her encouragement, support and perceptive comments at every stage of the research and writing.

TABLE OF CONTENTS

PREFACE

To understand what it is like to grow up with a life-threatening illness has been a personal and persistent curiosity of mine for a long time. Through a sociological study of cystic fibrosis I have achieved, at least partially, this understanding and it is towards communicating this achievement that this book is directed. The validity of my understanding is for the reader to decide.

AUTHOR'S NOTE

In order to preserve confidentiality,
the names of individuals, institutions
and organisations mentioned in this book
are fictitious.

TOWARDS A SOCIOLOGY OF GROWING UP
WITH A LIFE-THREATENING ILLNESS

Humans have the tendency "to make that permanent which
is in its nature transient." So speculated Canon
Gilles, a wise twelfth century French cleric in Helen
Waddell's (1933:18) classic version of *Peter Abelard*.
If Gilles was alive today he would find confirmation
of his speculation in the efforts of twentieth century
medicine; here, challenges to the vulnerability of
human life are confronted boldly in efforts to
vanquish threats to human permanence. Simultaneously,
because of the finite nature of life, this medical
propensity is doomed to failure.

Perhaps medical failure is most poignant when children
die from chronic diseases such as cancer, muscular
dystrophy and cystic fibrosis; these are the three
commonest disorders from which young people die. Life
and death conspicuously compose the two-edged sword of
the lives of children growing up with incurable
diseases such as these. The purpose of this book is
to provide at least a partial understanding of what it
is like to grow up with such life-threatening diseases
by looking at children and young adults with cystic
fibrosis.

CYSTIC FIBROSIS

Cystic fibrosis is an inherited disease affecting the exocrine glands which produce mucus, saliva and sweat; the most important abnormality is that mucus in various parts of the body is too thick. As a result, many tubules and spaces in the respiratory and digestive systems become obstructed. Left untreated, the working of the lungs is progressively compromised as shown by shortness of breath, fatigue and chest deformity. Infection ensues; colds turn into pneumonias and pneumonias fail to clear. In the digestive system, pancreatic ducts become obstructed and the pancreas atrophies; with insufficient pancreatic digestive enzyme secretion, difficulty in the absorption of food, particularly fat, results. The combination of poor absorption of food and protracted chest infection handicaps life chances considerably. In the past, few persons with cystic fibrosis lived beyond early childhood.

<u>Treatment</u>: Formerly, treatment consisted of pancreatic extracts with antibiotics and physiotherapy whenever a child with cystic fibrosis developed pneumonia. However, in 1956, intensive prophylactic therapy was started in Cleveland, Ohio, and has been taken up in whole or in part by many other child health centres.

This preventative therapy for the lungs includes:

1. physiotherapy - postural drainage of all main segments of the lungs, done twice daily in the home by the "parent(s)";

2. inhalation therapy - of substances which loosen mucus, used prior to physiotherapy;

3. antibiotics - for infection, given orally or nebulised into the lungs; and

4. immunisations - particularly against measles.

For the pancreas this therapy most frequently involves:

1. diet - fat restriction and the addition of unusual carbohydrates and fat-soluble vitamins; and

2. pancreatic extract - to supplement the enzyme secretion.

(Mearns, 1970: Holsclaw, 1970; Cook *et al.* 1959; Huang, 1972; Spock *et al.*, 1967; Kulczycki and Shwachman, 1958; Anderson, 1978; Doyle, 1959; Tecklin and Holsclaw, 1973; and Pryor *et al.*, 1979).

<u>Prognosis</u>: While prophylactic therapy is very demanding on parents and affected children, the latter's prognosis has improved remarkably (Shwachman *et al*., 1965; Anderson and Goodchild, 1976; and Anderson 1978). The most fortunate are reaching 30-plus years, with minimal embarrassing symptoms and deformities. However, the grim consequence is that many sufferers of cystic fibrosis survive childhood only to succumb in adolescence; growth failure occurs and chest infections become irradicable, eventuating in death.

<u>Incidence and Genetics</u>: Cystic fibrosis is the commonest hereditary disease among caucasians; its incidence is less common among other racial groups. One child in approximately every 1,600 white live births has the disease; approximately 2,000 new cases occur annually in the United States, 400 in the United Kingdom and nearly 100 in Australia (Anderson, 1978; Anderson and Goodchild, 1976; and Danks *et al*., 1965). The gene frequency is 1:20, and both parents of affected children must carry the cystic fibrosis gene. Thus, the probability of two carriers mating is 1:400; the chance of their children having the disease is 1:4 (McCrae *et al*., 1973). A female with cystic fibrosis has a 1:20 chance of mating with a carrier; if she does their children will have a 1:2 chance of being affected. Males with cystic fibrosis are infertile because their seminiferous tubules are

obstructed with mucus. While there is a great deal of promising research being done, at present the carrier state cannot be detected nor can the condition be diagnosed early in pregnancy (Pines, 1978; Anderson, 1978; and Anderson and Goodchild, 1976).

Symptoms and Diagnosis: Symptoms of cystic fibrosis include: frequent foul-smelling stools, growth failure, ravenous appetite, low physical stamina, persistent cough with excessive amounts of mucus, recurrent respiratory infections, clubbing of the fingers and excessive sweating. Bowel obstruction and nasal polyps may also occur.

Initially, cystic fibrosis is often confused with other diseases because of similar symptoms. The final diagnosis of cystic fibrosis is aided by a "sweat test": finding elevated sodium and chloride levels in the sweat (cf. Anderson and Goodchild, 1976).

It is within this context that children grow up with cystic fibrosis and from which much of the social science literature on the disease proceeds.

THE SOCIAL SCIENCE LITERATURE ON CYSTIC FIBROSIS

In the social science literature, discussion commonly centres on the economic, social and psychological problems posed by the disease and its therapy. There is a series of articles on the economic burden shouldered by families with affected children (Turk, 1964; Kulczycki, 1970; McCollum, 1971; and Beveridge and Lykke, 1973). These articles end with suitable remarks about the need to alleviate this burden, the advantages of a national health system and the possibilities of welfare capitalism mitigating financial stress.

There are research attempts to provide an understanding of the social problems associated with the disease. Here the standard focus is on the family coping with the daily drudge of prophylactic therapy, the uncertainties and stigma of genetics, sibling rivalry and marital breakdown and a brief discussion on "death in the family" (Allan et al., 1973; McCollom and Gibson, 1970; Burton, 1975; McCrae et al. 1973; Mikkelsen et al., 1978; and Meyerowitz and Kaplan, 1967). The conclusion reached is that stress could strengthen family ties but more commonly, the social problems posed by cystic fibrosis serve to detract from, rather than contribute to, family life.

Furthermore in the literature there are discussions on the psychological problems created by the disease with emphasis on parental rejection or over-protection of the affected child, and the afflicted adolescent's anxieties, depressions and rebellions about "being different" and "being treated differently" (Lawler et al, 1966; Cummings et al., 1966; Kulczycki et al, 1969; Batten, 1966; Edwards, 1966; Spock and Stedman, 1966; Pinkerton, 1969; Teicher, 1969; Tropauer et al., 1970; and Matthews et al, 1969).

6

Finally, ways to facilitate compliance and utilization of therapy are presented (Frydman, 1980).

This literature is good; it is neat and concise, yields systematic and comparable findings and has the support of medical officialdom. More importantly, for the purpose of this book, the literature clearly illustrates that cystic fibrosis is more than a disease: a biological entity having singular cause, effect and treatment. It is an illness having extraordinary social and psychological ramifications for afflicted persons and their families, friends and acquaintances which must be taken into account if the pathology is to be managed. However, essential as this contribution is, a sociological understanding of what it is like to grow up with cystic fibrosis is not reached. This is because the literature is oriented towards what Straus (1951) calls the "sociology *in* medicine" perspective: research directly applicable to patient care and the solving of health-related problems; it belongs to the realm of medical not sociological inquiry (Dingwall, 1976).

In order to achieve the understanding of what it is like to grow up with cystic fibrosis, or any other life-threatening illness, it is necessary to adopt a "sociology *of* medicine" perspective and undertake genuine field research whereby we look, listen and feel with these people; to be as Twaddle (1982) and align oneself with the patient's point of view. However, this literature and many medical sociology textbooks do not encourage such field research;

7

rather, they encourage highly systematic survey and experimental designs. The reason for this deficiency is not hard to find. As with Polsky's (1971) hustlers and beats, field research of the ill requires, among other things, giving up any and every kind of social work orientation and assumption. With respect to sociologists, in their struggles to be accepted into the healing world, many have joined forces with social workers under the position of "applied sociology" or "action research". Some of these sociologists have come to this position from mistaken conceptions of the nature of sociological understanding, others from a genuine concern to be of help to the sick, and others from an appraisal of how to achieve some status within the medical empire's halo. Whatever the motive, surely they are wrong to confuse sociology with social work and, although the use of survey and experimental research does not confuse the two necessarily, within the medical context they seem to have that propensity.

It is from this stance that the methodology of the present research proceeds.

METHODOLOGY

For five years primarily in parts of the United States and Australia, I have pursued my curiosity to understand what it is like to grow up with a life-threatening disease. During 1978 and 1979 these efforts were more research oriented: I talked with children and young adults who had cystic fibrosis; I talked with families of affected children and families who had lost children with cystic fibrosis; I talked with nearly anyone who was willing to talk about cystic fibrosis including paediatricians, nurses, social workers, dietitians, pharmacists, bio-medical scientists, teachers, parents, brothers and sisters, aunts and uncles, grandparents, my colleagues and students. Conversations took place in hospitals, clinics, offices, homes, aeroplanes, milk bars and schools. Furthermore, I participated in home physio-therapy sessions, sat in on various clinical discussions and briefings and reviewed numerous newsletters of cystic fibrosis associations and chapters.

The sample cannot be considered representative since only availability and network sampling techniques were employed. The non-representative nature of the sample, however, is not a major drawback since the analysis does not focus on characteristic traits of people with the disease or upon the problems and life events they typically face; rather, the focus is upon the cultural theme which emerges while children grow up with cystic fibrosis.

Cultural themes are learned and shared logic that "make sense" out of what Goffman (1961) calls "focussed gatherings". I prefer the term "focussed network of relationships"; I think focussed network captures the idea of a set of dispersed persons in a variety of social positions engrossed in a common flow of activity and relating to one another in terms of that flow more adequately than does Goffman's term.

Through diverse and sensitive tapping into a focussed network, a researcher learns and shares its cultural theme, its logic, that makes life in the network understandable.

Persons afflicted with cystic fibrosis or, in their own terms cystics, cystic fibrotics or CFs, grow up within the cystic fibrosis network of relationships. For personal reasons and through the wide variety of fortuitous avenues made available to me through friends, relatives and acquaintances, I have had the opportunity to gain entry into this network and learn and share its cultural theme - the logic through which an understanding of what it is like to grow up with the disease is obtained.

Articulating this logic, conceptualising this understanding and generalising the results of these efforts to other life-threatening illnesses has pre-occupied me from 1980 through most of 1982. Along these lines drafts of my written thoughts were circulated to people in medicine and in the social sciences; I talked about my ideas at sociology conferences and congresses from Australia to Mexico. The result of all this is that while there are many significant differences between children growing up with the variety of life-threatening illnesses, there seem to be some very significant similarities. It is the similarities that this book is about.

What I say in this book is my interpretation of my experiences, correspondence and conversations.

Obviously, I find value in these interpretations but it is important to note that the book itself does not capture the actual reality of growing up with a life-threatening illness; no book could. This book is simply my understanding of what it is like to grow up with a life-threatening illness.

GROWING UP WITH A LIFE-THREATENING ILLNESS

The "ceremonial order of the clinic" (Strong, 1979) may be characterised as an exchange of faith for hope. Within the clinic faith is the extent to which an ill person relies upon or trusts a medical person for knowledge about an ailment and its treatment; hope is the extent to which an ill person desires or expects to live a full, healthy life.

Strong's study is a good example of sociological field work: sensitive and full of insight. Yet, his focus on the clinic is unnecessarily "medicocentric"; this criticism is pertinent particularly for chronic diseases and physical and mental impairments where not only medical and para-medical but also familial and para-familial people are involved in therapy. Medical and para-medical personnel largely consist of doctors, nurses, physiotherapists, dietitians and social workers; familial and para-familial people include family, close friends, school teachers, employers and directors of swimming, scouting and other recreational activities. The common defining characteristics of these people are varying degrees of intimacy with the afflicted person and knowledge about the disease and its treatment. Thus, a more productive approach for the purpose of this study may be to focus on the ceremonial order of the therapeutic network in its broadest sense.

Medical and familial people may be labelled "insiders" in contrast to "outsiders" who lack this intimacy and knowledge. It is not uncommon to avoid and conceal this intimacy and knowledge with outsiders, and, for people growing up with a life-threatening illness, such concealment is frequently a necessary and regular part of life; disclosure makes an outsider an insider and thereby necessitates a faith/hope exchange. However, people, circumstances and disease symptoms prohibit complete control over intimacy and knowledge; medical personnel and families move, siblings are not discreet, age forces young people to shift from children's to adult hospitals and physical needs, symptoms and disabilities, as well as compliances with a medical regime, among other factors, put privacy at a premium and precariously promote new faith/hope exchanges.

In this chapter I try to present children growing up with life-threatening illnesses, their manipulations of intimacy and knowledge with outsiders and their faith/hope exchanges with insiders from their point of view. In other words, the material below avoids a "social problem" focus, a focus which predominates in the social science literature on children growing up with life-threatening illnesses. In so far as I treat the problems associated with such illnesses, they are not the problems the child creates for others, such as sibling rivalry, marital friction, economic burden and the difficulties with compliance and utilisation of therapy. Rather, I treat the problems others create for these children as they pursue hope and offer faith within their therapeutic network of relationships.

FAITH AND HOPE

For children growing up with a life-threatening illness there are many characteristic traits of faith, from trust in revealing symptoms or deformities, possible genetic implications, treatment and prognosis to reliance upon others for diet, medication, physio-therapy or supportive devices; there are many charac-teristic traits of hope from recreational, education and occupational activities to marriage and procrea-tional plans. As a result of these numerous characteristics, it is not difficult to understand the common notion that no two afflicted children are ever alike. In many ways it is this belief in the uniqueness of each child's case that makes hope and faith, even in the face of irrefutable statistical evidence to the contrary, possible within the thera-peutic network. Nevertheless, when a child is diagnosed as having a life-threatening illness, most often a sequence of interlocking steps, similar to Roth's (1963) "bench marks" in the career of tubercu-losis patients, is initiated: (1) introducing therapy; (2) selecting a doctor; (3) going to clincis; and (4) making changes as the child grows older. This sequence of interlocking steps is a generalised complex process occurring throughout a child's life; health crises and hospitalisations may intervene at any stage in this process as may the termination of life. Furthermore, the outsider is an ubiquitous feature in this sequence. There are other significant aspects to the life of a child growing up with a life-threatening illness, but it is largely within this context that the ceremonial order of the network occurs.

1. Introducing Therapy

The ceremonial exchange develops initially as a spontaneous attempt to cope with the realisation that, unlike other children whose lives seem "permanent", the lives of children with life-threatening illnesses seem highly "transient". The decision to initiate therapy may be viewed as an attempt to make permanent that which appears transient; while biological factors are taken into account, the decision not to introduce therapy is based on viewing this attempt as futile.

For example, a paediatrician at a children's hospital did not introduce the time-consuming in-the-home daily medical regime for a particular baby diagnosed as having cystic fibrosis. Biological factors alone were not the reason: the mother was in her early teens and living with her younger sister. While keeping weekly checks on the baby's condition and making sure the baby was not in pain, rigorous prophylactic therapy was not initiated. The doctor regarded the situation as hopeless; the baby died in a few weeks.

The important point here is that right from the start social as well as biological factors are taken into account in the treatment of children growing up with life-threatening illnesses. For all people in the therapeutic network, afflicted children and medical and familial people, social factors are not merely the "pudding" of life, but, along with biology, are the very stuff of life.

Upon initiating therapy, the ceremonial order of the network commences. After commencement, selection of an appropriate doctor occurs.

2. Selecting a Doctor

The faith/hope exchange, which begins as a spontaneous attempt to cope, becomes entrenched and forms the basis upon which families of children with life-threatening illnesses select their doctor. The concern here is twofold: (1) selecting a specialist and (2) selecting a general practitioner. Only in the larger urban areas is it possible to have a choice amongst specialists in cystic fibrosis, muscular dystrophy or cancer. Even in large cities, selection is frequently limited; in the United States there is a highly organised network of local cystic fibrosis centres usually directed by a pulmonary or gastro-enterological paediatrician. In rural areas, and very often in cities, families select a general practitioner for the care of their afflicted child. Whenever selection occurs, it does not seem to be based upon "bedside manner" or factors such as time spent in the waiting room. Rather as Bury (1982) notes, families search for a doctor with apparent complete medical knowledge: "a doctor one can trust". Unfortunately, the treatment of cystic fibrosis is partially based upon "trial-and-error" with respect to drugs and diet. A thorough doctor may make frequent changes in the medical regime to maximise the care of growing children; this practice may undermine trust unless the changes are carefully explained to the family.

After an appropriate doctor is selected, the child starts a practice which in one form or another, will continue for his or her life time: going to clinics.

3. Going to Clinics

Fortnightly, monthly or bi-monthly, mothers, some fathers and a few entire families escort their ill children to a clinic. Here, the child's treatment and progress are assessed and alterations in dosages and regimes are made; thorough physiotherapies may be completed, dietitians, social workers and visiting nurses offer their services and consultation with his or her paediatrician occurs. Simultaneously, the clinic serves as an important occasion for reviewing the faith paid and the hope received.

This faith/hope review often serves to put (1) the clinic and (2) the daily home therapy in a positive light. For ease of administration, usually the clinics are structured such that they become endurance tests for the families. That is, all patients are booked in at the same time rather than staggered. Slowly, each person is seen by the relevant medical and para-medical personnel. It is an ordeal but the families wait, look around at each other and more often than not conclude that they are lucky; it seems that there are always children worse off then theirs. The daily task of performing prophylactic therapy seems worth it and the clinic becomes a venue where hope is nurtured and faith is renewed.

While this balancing of faith with hope continues, the children grow older and changes other than in drugs or diet occur. One such significant social change which gradually emerges is the child's participation in the exchange process.

4. Making Changes as the Child Grows Older

Children learn the exchange process from their parents; in other words, what developed initially as an attempt to cope with the realisation that their child's life is highly transient and became entrenched as the means to obtain its permanence, is appropriated as the *modus operandi* by the adolescent.

Allen *et al*. (1974), Batten (1966), Matthews *et al* (1969), Teicher (1969) and Shwachman *et al*. (1965) posit that adolescence is especially fraught with change and difficulty for the cystic; uncertainty of prognosis, employment prospects and socially embar-rassing symptoms plague the adolescent and make full appropriation of the faith/hope exchange a herculean task. The transfer from child health care services to health provisions for total care as an adult further jeopardises their favourable faith for hope exchange. For example, a physiotherapist reports that a teenage cystic died because she was too frightened to go to an adult hospital. She was admitted very sick to the children's hospital and when told that she had to go to the adult hospital she stopped talking and died within the week.

Although this physiotherapist may be overstating the effect transfer from child to adult health care services may have, there is an increasing number of adults with cystic fibrosis; besides the need to implement appropriate social and medical provisions for the care of adult cystics, it is imperative that their transition from child to adult facilities be done in such a way so as to minimize any detrimental effects to the delicate faith/hope balance.

Outsiders

Throughout this sequence of stages is the outsider. As with Goffman's (1963) stigmatised people, initial intimacy with children and knowledge about their life-threatening illness and treatment may originate an unfavourable faith/hope exchange; concealment, however, may be impossible.

For example, initially parents and older siblings may conceal the hereditary nature of an illness.

Engagements, marriages and future pregnancies for all in the family however, would prohibit concealment, or what Edgerton (1967) calls a "benevolent conspiracy", and prescribe a faith/hope exchange: a frequently precarious exchange for the cystic, his family and the outsider.

School also occasions the cystic and outsiders to be together. Coughs, low physical stamina, increased appetite, frequent bowel actions, numerous days absence due to respiratory infections, and the need for a myriad of antibiotic and pancreatic extract tablets circumscribe attempts at total concealment. While the cystic gives faith, his expectation for hope is frequently frustrated by teachers, who unknowingly find it difficult to render hope to a child with a short life expectation. Coupled with possible peer isolation, the probability of a favourable faith/hope exchange is questionable.

Genetics and the short life expectancy further prohibit concealing the disease from young adult cystics' dates and prospective spouses; disclosing the disease, however, frequently condemns the young cystic, or other similarly ill adolescent, to isolation. For example, Gill, an 18 year old "master of dress", as described by her doctor, is already resigned to a lonely adult life; she argues that no one wants to go out with her because she has cystic fibrosis. It should be noted however, that isolation is not inevitable. Rewarding friendships and happy marriages happen.

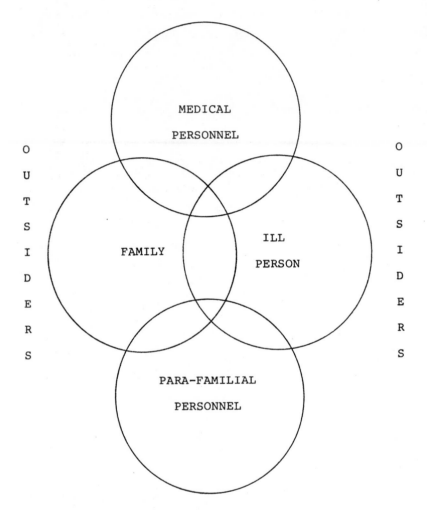

O
U
T
S
I
D
E
R
S

O
U
T
S
I
D
E
R
S

MEDICAL

PERSONNEL

FAMILY

ILL

PERSON

PARA-FAMILIAL

PERSONNEL

Figure 1.   THE THERAPEUTIC NETWORK OF RELATIONSHIPS

Health Crisis, Hospitalisation and the Termination of Therapy and Life

The fatal outcome usually begins with a health crisis and proceeds to hospitalisation, the termination of therapy and, eventually, of life. Throughout this process is a gradual withdrawal of faith and hope from the cystic fibrosis network. A chief physiotherapist at a children's hospital elucidates this process:

> There is a kind of unwritten law that if a child like that (dying cystic fibrotic) comes into hospital there's a little sort of conference goes on with people saying that, "well, he is going to die very shortly", you know, within a matter of 3 or 4 days. Well then again, people have a little think and they say, "we will make him comfortable - that's all". And that means things like oxygen, medications which make life a bit happy, every sort of comfort in what they want to eat or drink they can indulge in, you know. If they want champagne at midnight, somebody will buzz off and get it; but mostly, of course, they're too ill to want this sort of thing. There are no dramatics, especially these days; that has got much better. Then to stop the child and the parents (although the parents should be aware - people have failed if the parents aren't aware that this child will die very shortly) from despair, we don't withdraw all treatment and therapy from the patient all at once, because usually by the time the child reaches that age they've got to know and got used to us. And they regard us as friends whom they have a great deal of trust in. Even if we just visit and only pat them gently on the back and go to talk to them a few minutes a day, it satisfies their sort of whatever they are looking for - er - you know. So a physiotherapist on the ward, who knows the child, will pop along perhaps four

times a day and have a chat and nominal
treatment but, you know, it's just a
gesture, until they no longer want to see us
and say "go away" or something; then we stop
and they lose consciousness.

Another case which illustrates this faith/hope withdrawal further may be paraphrased in the following
manner:

A young teenage boy with cystic fibrosis was
admitted to hospital. His doctor instructed
us to give him the works. I (a physiotherapist) was on duty the whole of that weekend
and I was told to see that this child had
physio and the full treatment every four
hours and try to keep his chest clear. He
was in an oxygen tent, very unco-operative
with us. The whole thing was really
appalling. So I rang his doctor up and
said, "I'm sorry but I'm not going to go on
treating him". "Oh yes, you must. You
must. We must give these parents who sit
beside the children's beds hope that we
haven't abandoned them. We mustn't show
them we've given up", (the boy's doctor
replied). Now his parents were divorced and
one was in Sydney and the other in London.
He was entrusted to a rich aunt here. So I
said to him (the boy's doctor) "Look he's
going to die, isn't he, very shortly?"
"Yes, yes, but it wouldn't do not to treat
him" (the boy's doctor replied). So I
thought about it a bit and it was on an
Easter Sunday afternoon, so I rang up Dr.
G---, our medical director at home and I
said, "I'm sorry to disturb you but I just
told Dr. S--- (the boy's doctor) that I will
not do anything about his case". I
described it all to him. "So if you have
any repercussions, I'm sorry, but that's how
it is." He said, "O.K., that's fine." The
child died at 4 o'clock that afternoon or
something like that. The whole thing
appalling; this vigorous postural drainage

that was requested was macabre. He knew he
was dying and that we couldn't do anything
about it. He didn't want to be bothered by
physios. We couldn't do anything for him.

CONCLUSION

Intensive therapy, although a requisite, does not
ensure a full, healthy life for a child growing up
with cystic fibrosis or with muscular dystrophy or
cancer. Rather, the effects of prophylactic therapy
may be viewed as mediated through an exchange of
symbols - meanings and definitions. This exchange is
exceptionally complex, since its relevant symbols are
faith and hope; symbols frequently not having empiri-
cal referents (Vernon, 1978).

Clearly, the life experiences of children with these
life-threatening illnesses generally endorse symbols
of hope; for example, fear of frustrated hope
expectations maintains the cystic in a cocoon of
isolation from outsiders. On the other hand, cystics
show a sensitivity towards insiders' needs for faith;
lack of faith is at times responsible for doctors
eschewing their patients and parents their children.
In other words, children with life-threatening illnesses need the hope medical and familial people
consign and these insiders need the faith the children
award. This exchange permits the children, their
families and medical personnel to devote themselves to
the rigorous demands of prophylactic therapy by
ameliorating the certain uncertainty: the inevitability of an early death.

The functional necessity for faith and hope within the therapeutic network of relationships however, does not ensure their presence. Their reality is constantly threatened by the uncertainties underlying the disease. Chapter 3 discusses the neutralisation of these uncertainties.

TECHNIQUES OF NEUTRALISATION

The ceremonial order of the clinic or network is a precarious reality. It is constantly threatened by the uncertainties underlying the epidemiology of the disease; inconclusive answers to questions of etiology, treatment and prognosis undermine trust and sabotage expectations (cf. Berger and Luckman, 1967; and Berger, 1969).

For those growing up with a life-threatening illness, faith and hope would seem to be implausible realities within their networks. However, neither the inevitability of an early death nor the epidemiological uncertainties of cystic fibrosis ordinarily deter the exchange of faith and hope. Cystics and their families typically trust in their prophylactic therapy and in the people who help administer it; typically, a full healthy life is expected for the cystic child and, accordingly, recreational, educational, occupational and even marital plans are made. In short, there is a process of central importance at work within the cystic fibrosis network, and apparently in the therapeutic networks of children growing up with other life-threatening illnesses that serves to support the "swaying edifice" of faith and hope. This is the process of neutralisation.

Neutralisation is the process whereby confrontation with the epidemiological questions of an illness is deflected; the uncertainties that serve to check or inhibit faith and hope are rendered inoperative and the people within the therapeutic network of relation-ships are free to engage in their exchange without serious threats to its currency.

It is the purpose of this chapter to capture the process of neutralisation within the cystic fibrosis therapeutic network.

THE PROCESS OF NEUTRALISATION

With cystic fibrosis there are five significant uncertainties which undermine faith and hope. These are:

1. etiology - the cause of cystic fibrosis is unknown;

2. genetics - cystic fibrosis cannot be diagnosed early in pregnancy nor can the carrier state be detected;

3. treatment - type of diet and the value and dosages of select tablets among other factors in the treatment of cystic fibrosis, are controversial;

4. societal reaction - this little known, inherited and, at times, difficult-to-conceal disease fre-quently stigmatises the child and family; and

5. life expectancy - the life of a person with cystic fibrosis is shortened but indeterminate ranging from a few days to thirty-plus years. It is by neutralising these uncertainties that faith and hope are made secure.

This process of neutralisation is similar to that of Sykes and Matza (1957). In analysing the process within the cystic fibrosis network, it is convenient to divide it into five major techniques. These are:

1. the modification of the question;

2. the promise of research;

3. the uniqueness of each case;

4. the comparison with others; and

5. the lack of an alternative to therapy.

Each technique addresses a particular uncertainty underlying cystic fibrosis.

1. Modification of the Question

In so far as an epidemiological question can be modified to elicit certitude, the effectiveness of uncertainty in undermining faith and hope is sharply reduced. The etiological question readily lends itself to this technique of neutralisation.

The basis of this affinity lies in the prediagnostic etiological question asked and answered. The pre-diagnostic query concerns the etiology of symptoms, not the disease.

> "Patty ate and ate and never gained weight."
> - Mother of a 3 year old cystic girl.

> "Tom used to cough and cough all night."
> - Father of a 3 year old cystic boy.

> "Barbara's stools were foul-smelling."
> - Mother of a 4 year old cystic girl.

Typically, there is a great deal of difficulty in securing an answer to explain these symptoms. Asthma, allergies, hereditary thinness and "common infant behaviour" are frequent diagnoses. This inaccuracy jeopardises faith in medical knowledge and shatters hope for the survival of the child. Uncertainty ends with the diagnosis of cystic fibrosis; the diagnosis credibly explains the ravenous appetite, minimum weight-gain, racking cough and foul-smelling stools. While deeply hurt, parents feel a sense of relief from the uncertainties underlying this etiological quest (Mikkelsen *et al.*, 1978). When correctly diagnosed, the possibility of alleviating the symptoms through therapy exists. As the symptoms are controlled, faith in cystic fibrosis therapy and in medical personnel commences; simultaneously, as the child responds to treatment, hope is restored.

In order to secure faith and hope, further etiological questions are not broached. The question of the etiology of cystic fibrosis is modified; the cystic fibrosis network moves on to asking and providing credible answers to questions of prevention and contagion.

"Nothing parents do directly causes cystic fibrosis." Nevertheless, parents often assume responsibility for their child's disease. With various degrees of severity and regularity, uncertainty about inadequate diet during pregnancy, faulty sperm and the wrath of God for previous sins arises; personal, sexual and marital problems frequently follow. Dietitians, genetic counsellors, religious directors and particularly parents of other cystic children quieten these uncertainties. "Nothing parents do directly causes cystic fibrosis. But it takes one of us to convince another ..." - the father of a boy with cystic fibrosis states.

Neither is cystic fibrosis communicable; it is transmitted genetically. However, the possibility of contagion is a frequent query of school teachers, as well as of other para-familial personnel. The cystic fibrosis network arms parents with brochures graphically depicting the genetic transmission of cystic fibrosis; armouries of official pamphlets lend credence to parental answers.

As a technique of neutralisation, the modification of the etiological question does more than render

inoperative uncertainties that undermine faith and
hope. It enables positive answers to arise in the
light of an otherwise bleak diagnosis. Questions of
responsibility and of the need for quarantine are
credibly answered; feelings of guilt and fears of
contagion need not maintain the cystic and his family
in a cocoon of isolation. Parents and children are to
"get on with the business of living."

"Getting on with the business of living is what we are
all about", a nurse reports. This business rarely
includes directly questioning the etiology of cystic
fibrosis. When it does, paediatricians readily modify
the question: "Did you know that the cause of most
diseases is unknown? The important thing is to keep
the child alive and healthy."

It is not the reason for modifying the etiology
question that is of concern here, but its function of
deflecting uncertainty in medical knowledge (cf.
Frank, 1979). By modifying this question, further
confrontation between medical uncertainty and the
precarious realities of faith and hope is avoided.

2. The Promise of Research

The second technique of neutralisation centres on the
uncertainties of having a baby with cystic fibrosis.
Research efforts into cystic fibrosis address these
uncertainties: detecting the carrier state and
diagnosing the disease early in pregnancy.

The ability to detect the carrier state enables a couple who are both carriers to consider the alternatives of artificial insemination by donor rather than risk having an affected child. The ability to diagnose *in utero* in early pregnancy by, for example, examining amniotic fluid enables parents to have the option of terminating an affected pregnancy.

However, within the network, failure turns on the question of time: "It is only a matter of time before we have success here," a paediatrician assures staff and patients.

This assurance works. In recent years, fewer parents with cystic children risk further pregnancies except by artificial insemination by donor; more siblings postpone pregnancy. Young people feel confident that medical research will keep its promise.

The alternatives (i.e. termination of affected pregnancies and artificial insemination by donor) made possible through pre-natal diagnosis and detection of the carrier state will need to be elucidated to these young people. With sensitive elucidation of the alternatives, when they become realities, medical research becomes another gesture of the healer's art (Cassell, 1978).

3. The Uniqueness of Each Case

The uncertainty arising from different treatment may be neutralised by an insistence that each case of cystic fibrosis is unique and must be treated as such by the medical personnel concerned. Thus, differences are not really differences; rather, each is the best treatment in the light of singular circumstances.

As Sykes and Matza (1957) would say, by a "subtle alchemy" medical personnel prescribe the best combination of enzymes, diets, vitamins and physiotherapy for each patient. Certainty on the proper dosages of Viokase, Pancreatin or Cotazyme B is obvious; the correct amount of fatty, fried and starchy foods is readily calculable; controversies over the value of Pentavite, Abidec, Vidaylin and vitamin E preparations are non-existent; idiosyncracies over the use of nebulization mixtures and mist-tent therapy are figments of the imagination.

This technique of neutralisation begins with the pamphlets parents receive when their child is diagnosed cystic fibrotic. For example, a typical pamphlet reads:

> When visiting the hospital, or otherwise meeting with parents of children with cystic fibrosis, it is most important not to compare differences in the methods by which the patient is being treated. Each case of cystic fibrosis is approached as being quite individual, and must be treated as such by the doctors concerned.

Thus, differences amongst doctors in their treatment of cystic fibrosis are transformed into individualised regimes to meet the uniqueness of each case.

The concern here is not to deny the uniqueness of each case. The concern is to show that uncertainty, resulting from the differences in cystic fibrosis therapy, is neutralised by an insistence on the uniqueness of each case.

4. The Comparison with Others

A fourth technique of neutralisation involves a comparison with less fortunate others. The cystic fibrosis network shifts the focus of the stigma from this little-known, hereditary and difficult to conceal disease to the more obvious misfortunes of people who are mentally retarded, spastic or who have spina bifida (Allan et al. 1974; and DeJong, 1980).

That is, whenever cystics and their families cannot conceal the disease from outsiders, they must manage the "identity uncertainties" disclosure provokes (Goffman, 1959, 1963, 1967; Davis, 1961; Davis 1973; Voysey, 1972; and Strauss, 1959). Errors and misconceptions about the disease are never-ending; feelings of being the "unclean" part of the family are commonly reported; coughs, frequent and foul-smelling bowel actions, low physical stamina and numerous days absence from school subject children to ridicule, isolation and hostility from siblings, peers and directors of educational and recreational activities.

As do Gussow and Tracy's (1968) "lepers", the cystic fibrosis network develops a "stigma theory" that may not disavow their imputed inferiority but does enable the condition to be more palatable to them. The comparison with others less fortunate than themselves is such a stigma theory; it is a consciously-created perspective within the cystic fibrosis network which functions to neutralise the uncertainties about self brought about when concealment is not possible in interpersonal encounters (Glaser and Strauss, 1964).

The validity of their theory is not as important as its function in deflecting self-doubts arising from societal reaction to this little-known, hereditary and difficult to conceal disease. By means of this technique of neutralisation, the cystic fibrosis network, in effect, has changed the focus of the stigma from these aspects of the disease to the greater misfortunes of others; by focusing on others, the uncertainties underlying the cystic and his family's sense of identity are more easily lost to view.

5. The Lack of an Alternative to Therapy

Allan *et al*. (1974) report that denial of the inevit-able prognosis is the easiest response cystics and their families can make; Burton (1975) argues that commonly the response to a limited future is day-to-day resignation. However, neither the denial of the inevitable prognosis nor day-to-day resignation to a limited future neutralises the uncertainties underlying a shortened but indeterminate life expectancy (Davis, 1960; and Kubler-Ross, 1978).

Premature death is a too obvious reality of the cystic fibrosis network to be denied; attempts at its postponement are too poignant a reality for resignation to be a possibility.

Not that the cystic fibrosis network necessarily repudiates denial or resignation. Rather, the network is caught up in a logic of expediency that inadvertently jettisons these defence mechanisms in order to hold in abeyance the ultimate irrationality that threatens their faith/hope exchange: the inevitability of an early death.

In contrast to the elderly, the terminally ill child or young adult is a rarity. Because of their rarity, credible reasons to "make sense" out of premature death do not exist (Baker, 1978; and Parker and Mauger, 1979); denial and resignation are the initial responses. However, while denial and resignation may be the earliest modes of adaptation, they do little to safeguard the faith and hope necessary for devotion to the expediency of prophylactic therapy.

Furthermore, the medical world is impotent. Infectious diseases are curable, but prolonging a relatively healthy life is the best medical personnel can expect to achieve with cystic fibrosis. Often, inhibiting a slow, relentless decline is their task. Uncertainty abounds; an uncertainty that undermines devotion to the cystic fibrosis regime. For example, a former visiting nurse reports:

> I took care of Karen until she was 16, when she died with cystic fibrosis .... I doubt that it's worth it, but what are the alternatives? That's the thing.

That there is no other alternative is a belief that represents at least a tangential blow to the irrationality of the faith/hope exchange within the cystic fibrosis network. It is a credible logic that enables the network to suspend the uncertainties underlying a shortened, indeterminate life span and to devote themselves to the rigours of cystic fibrosis therapy (cf. Berger and Kellner, 1970; and Glaser and Strauss, 1968).

CONCLUSION

The techniques of neutralisation may not be powerful enough to shield fully the people in the cystic fibrosis network from the forces of uncertainty underlying the epidemiological questions of cystic fibrosis. Nevertheless, the techniques of neutralisation are critical in lessening the uncertainties that undermine the precarious realities of faith and hope within the network.

In the last resort, the cystic fibrosis network and possibly networks for children suffering from other life-threatening illnesses band together to forestall an early death through compliance with therapy. Ultimately, the success of the techniques is to be judged by the tenacity with which the people in the network devote themselves to complying with this therapy. The following chapter presents an analysis of this compliance.

4

COMPLYING WITH THERAPY

For persons growing up with a life-threatening illness, compliance with an intensive medical regime is a continually emerging process of their very existence.

While not negating its valuable contributions, the literature on compliance with medical care seems to ignore its emergent nature. Rather, by and large, the literature either focuses on determining factors responsible for poor compliance, such as characteristics of patients, regimes and illnesses, or it attempts to find social-psychological variables that would motivate compliance such as health beliefs in the seriousness of the disease and the efficacy of care or more effective communication patterns between health care providers and patients (Becker and Maiman, 1975 and 1980; Mitchell, 1974; Marston, 1970; Frydman, 1980; Strauss and Glaser, 1975; Sackett and Haynes, 1976; Stone, 1979; McKercher and Rucker, 1977; Davis, 1968; Davis and Eichhorn, 1963; and Charney, 1972).

I think that this literature provides too mechanistic a view of compliance, at least for children with life-threatening illnesses. The former type of literature generally focuses on factors neither alterable nor predictive due to their mutually contradictory nature; the later social-psychological type of literature seems "back-to-front" in accounting for compliance with therapy (Becker and Maiman, 1975; and Sackett and Haynes, 1976). That is, instead of compliant motivations leading to compliant behaviour, it seems to be the other way around; compliance in time produces its own motivations. In other words, from the spontaneous impulses, vague fears and vacillating hopes about the disease, its treatment and prognosis, therapy commences; through the changing social interpretations of the therapy, its techniques and effects, compliance, and non-compliance, emerge. In so far as there are motivations, these are not the geneses but the consequences of compliance.

In this chapter I try to present this emergent nature of compliance with therapy for persons afflicted with cystic fibrosis. With some modifications, the presentation is built around Howard Becker's (1953) three steps in becoming a marihuana user.

THE EMERGENT NATURE OF COMPLIANCE

Compliance with the regime of cystic fibrosis therapy necessitates:

1. learning its techniques;

2. learning to perceive its effects and

3. learning to enjoy its effects.

However, while these three steps are necessary, the development of a stable pattern of compliance is improbable; compliance is prescribed an emergent nature through powerful forces of social control that proscribe, or at least make inexpedient, stable compliance patterns. Inexpediency results in changes in interpretations of the therapy, its techniques and effects and may occur at any of these three steps and thus so may the emergence of non-compliance. This sequence of steps, forces of social control and changes in interpretations form a generalised complex process that initially affects the "parents" and family of the cystic child; later, this process affects the adolescent cystic. There are other significant aspects of utilising cystic fibrosis therapy but it is largely within this context that compliance emerges.

1. Learning the Techniques

Although cystic fibrosis therapy is highly systematic, ordinarily parents do not learn its techniques upon initial instructions; frequent visits to clinics as well as home-visits by nurses and physiotherapists are required. Furthermore, it is not uncommon to include several hospital stays in this early learning period.

There are three explanations of the apparent failure of the initial instructions:

1. the "trial-and-error" nature of establishing diets and tablet dosages;

2. the parents' psychological difficulties in doing physiotherapy on their infant; and

3. the parents' near overwhelming responsibility for the survival of their infant.

Apparently, one of the biggest problems in the initial establishment of therapy is setting the proper dosage of antibiotics and enzymes as well as vitamins and diet. The types and dosages of tablets vary for each child and the only way to establish the proper levels is by trial-and-error: continuously bringing the baby into the clinic to see how he or she is doing and try other "things" to see how they affect the child. It is not easy and the problem becomes compounded because the parents are worried during this time; they are not even used to the idea that their child has cystic fibrosis.

Parents are also worried about being able to do thorough physiotherapy on their infants because the necessary technique causes the child to cry, cough and turn red. Postural drainage of the lungs is not a pleasant task but it is necessary. The parents' sense of responsibility may be overwhelming because they realise that postural drainage is necessary for keeping their baby alive. Practical and social supports are often needed and visiting nurses, physiotherapists and members of cystic fibrosis chapters meet these needs.

Meeting these needs not only aids the "newtimers" to the cystic fibrosis network but also the "oldtimers". That is, support is mutually received and a better understanding of cystic fibrosis and its therapy is gained by teaching others.

It should be noted that due to changes in regime and in the life-cycle, learning the techniques of cystic fibrosis therapy is a continuous process. New knowledge about the disease and its treatment is frequently being disseminated and the requirements of an adolescent or young adult differ from those of a child. Formally, clinics and Cystic Fibrosis Associations attempt to keep people informed about these sorts of changes. Informally, an efficient device for this continual learning to occur is the teaching of the techniques of the therapy to others.

It is important to learn the techniques of the therapy in order for it to be effective. Only when it is effective is it possible to perceive the direct effects of the therapy and to distinguish these effects from its more indirect effects. Without such distinction, enjoyment of the effects is precluded and compliance regresses.

2.   Learning to Perceive the Effects

The direct effects of cystic fibrosis therapy include health, a promising prognosis and the mitigation of coughs, foul smells and the unpleasantness of postural drainage as well as the promotion of normal physical stamina and stature. The indirect effects include social responses to the treatment as well as to the disease (Zola, 1966); these responses may include sibling and peer rivalry, marital friction and divorce, and the psychological, physical and financial strains of coping daily with the time-consuming nature and intensity of the disease and treatment. In the minds of cystics and their families, it is not uncommon to confuse these two types of effects; if this confusion is not clarified, it is impossible to perceive and enjoy the direct effects of the therapy and compliance ceases.

As a necessary and regular part of medical care, social workers, dietitians, visiting nurses, physio-therapists and paediatricians attempt to encourage compliance by distinguishing these effects for their clients. The distinction requires that the direct effects be perceived and that their connection with the therapy be recognised by the cystic and his family; if indirect effects are perceived, it is imperative that the link with the therapy be obscured. Paraphrased excerpts from a pre-clinic briefing illustrate this necessary and regular part of medical care in encouraging compliance to emerge; these paraphrases also illustrate that doctors and other para-medical personnel do treat the whole person not just the biology and are concerned with illness and not just disease - a finding contrary to much social science fact or opinion:

Paediatrician: Er, let's see, now we'll also be seeing Anna K--, age 3 and 2 months. Last here two months ago ... Sputum has some blood in it; chest not good ... Hadn't gained weight ...

Dietitian: I'll talk with her (the mother) and see what Anna's been eating, but she never listens to me ...

Visiting Nurse: I've been to their home twice since they've been here. She's having problems. You know her husband left her last year? And I think she may be blaming it all on what's happened to her ... She's not facing her responsibilities and with work and wanting to go out she is quite frustrated ...

Physiotherapist: Does she do her physio?

Visiting Nurse: I have no idea. She says she does but I imagine its pretty sporadic ... I did it when I was there and there was lots of mucus and mess ...

Dietitian: What does she think is going to happen if she doesn't do what she is told!

Paediatrician: Hey, today I want all of you to try and really encourage her to really get into this thing. Tell her that once she is really into all this, all this strain Anna is causing will stop, and all her other problems she can then sort out. Besides, they have nothing to do really, with treating the baby.

Paediatrician: Christopher M is here today. He's 14 now ... we'll have to do something about that; can't let B-- (an adult hospital) get their hands on him yet ... Old Chris here, ain't doing so well. His chest is not clear and last time he was here he had a terrible cough. Perhaps a chest infection ...

Physiotherapist: I'm not surprised. His mother told me he fights with her to get out of doing postural drainage and he always forgets his tablets ...

Paediatrician: We'll have to find out why.

Social Worker: All teenagers go through this phase ...

Paediatrician: Yes, but this could be a fatal phase he won't get through ... His mother was always excelling in treating him ... It would be a shame to lose him now.

Social Worker: I'll talk with him, Doctor, but you really should. He likes you and, er, you know, he needs a male among us at his age to listen to ...

Paediatrician:	I'll do what I can. If it calls for banging him around the ears a bit I will ... He has to learn that it's not a disgrace to take tablets in school and out and to do physios ... I know it's hard but the kids would like him more not less if he stays healthy.

Paediatrician:	We're seeing Katherine Ann M--- today ... Here's a sad case. Her mother's pregnant .... The relationship fell through and there she is pregnant and blaming it and her loneliness on poor Katy, at least according to this report ...

Physiotherapist:	I know her mother, Helen, and will have a talk with her ... Tell her this fellow's leaving had nothing to do with Katherine and that Katy is so healthy due to all her hard work on her that it would be a pity to undo it all again now ...

During this research, I concluded that the lower the socio-economic status, the more difficult it is to distinguish the direct from indirect effects of therapy; compartmentalising the home therapy from other daily activities is more easily achieved in the larger houses of the more economically prosperous families; living in the same room with tables, sheets, nebulisers, tablets and possibly mechanical devices for chest physiotherapy, among other cystic fibrosis paraphernalia, not only makes it difficult to see where the direct effects end and the indirect effects begin but precipitates the indirect effects.

This inverse relationship between socio-economic status and compliance was frequently voiced by respondents. More frequently however, socio-economic status was reported to have a contradictory effect on compliance. That is, its positive relationship with the ease of distinguishing direct from indirect effects is inverted in learning to enjoy the direct effects; learning to enjoy these effects is essential for compliance to emerge as the central feature of a cystic fibrotic's life.

3. Learning to Enjoy the Effects

The higher the socio-economic status, the more difficult it is to enjoy the direct effects of cystic fibrosis therapy. Learning to enjoy these effects is a function of the degree of experience one has had with sickness, a poor prognosis, coughs, foul smells and unpleasant aspects of postural drainage, as well as with limited physical stamina and stature. Furthermore, enjoying the direct effects is relative to the expectations held for the therapy.

Cystic children from families of higher socio-economic status are less likely to have as high a degree of such experiences as are cystic children from families of lower socio-economic status. Furthermore, more economically prosperous families have higher expectations of cystic fibrosis therapy than do less economically prosperous families.

A consequence of learning to enjoy the direct effects of compliance with cystic fibrosis therapy is the development of compliant motivations. However, counter to these motivations are powerful forces of social control that proscribe, or at least make inexpedient, the development of stable compliance patterns and prescribe an emergent nature for compliance.

Social Control

Compliant motivations may be countered to the extent that cystics and their families find compliance inexpedient or believe that they will find it so. This real or presumed inexpediency arises from the fact or belief that if discovered with the disease or complying with its therapy, negative sanctions will be applied. For example, family members may fear rejection from spouse, dates and prospective spouses due to the genetic basis of the disease; adolescent cystics may fear rejection or hostility from peers, siblings and parents, school teachers and directors of scouting, swimming and other recreational activities due to "being different" or "being treated differently".

For the adolescent, some of this social control may break down in the course of complying with the therapy. That is, with the development of the direct effects of the therapy the cystic comes to realize that as long as he remains healthy (1) some peers need never discover he is "different" and (2) "differential treatment" may be minimised; coughs, low physical stamina, increased appetite, frequent bowel actions, numerous days absence from school due to respiratory infections and the need for a myriad of antibiotic and pancreatic extract tablets circumscribe attempts at concealing differences and promote fear of rejection and hostility; a school teacher exclaimed that "it is a pain ..." for her and for the other children to have Jill, a young unhealthy cystic child, in the classroom. Thus, the paediatrician from the pre-clinic briefing encourages compliance by saying ".... the kids would like him (Christopher) more, not less, if he stays healthy."

Similarly, as with Goffman's (1963) stigmatised people, due to fear and anxiety parents and older siblings may conceal the child's hereditary disease.

Such an environment does not encourage rigorous compliance; coupled with the physical and financial strains on the family, compliance is, at least, inexpedient.

Fear and anxiety result in real and presumed inexpediency when learning the techniques of the therapy as well as when perceiving and enjoying its direct effects; with each occurrence new interpretations of the therapy, its techniques and effects form, prescribing the emergent nature of compliance. Also, from these formations, non-compliance inevitably emerges.

Non-compliance

The inevitable emergence of non-compliance allows it to be dismissed as primarily a response to biological factors, " .... the progressive compromise of the lungs, poor absorption of food and the eventual chest infection must inevitably end in non-compliance" with cystic fibrosis therapy, a nurse posits. Of course there may be a biological state when compliance cannot benefit the cystic, but there are several reasons for rejecting this fact as the fundamental justification for dismissing non-compliance as primarily a response to biological factors.

One reason is that non-compliance is by no means unequivocally endorsed by families and medical personnel when, biologically, therapy cannot "cure" nor comfort very ill cystics. Much is said on the subject of euthanasia but, more often, are the exhortations "to keep trying" rather than "to let die" (cf. Sudnow, 1967; and Fox, 1976).

A second and more sociologically significant reason for refusing to accept a biological explanation for non-compliance is that this position leaves unexplained the intermittent non-compliance of healthy cystics. For example, young teenage healthy cystics frequently "forget" to take tablets, rebel against physiotherapy and cheat on diet. If a healthy cystic with a good prognosis fails to comply with therapy, surely non-compliance is more than a response to biology.

Another case is Beth. With racking cough and gasping breath she realises that she is dying and that family and medical personnel "unintentionally" are not encouraging compliance, yet she insists on having her tablets, physiotherapy and proper diet.

Such cases show that the reasons for the inevitable emergence of non-compliance will remain mysterious as long as it continues to be dismissed as a response to poor biology. A more productive approach begins with regarding non-compliance as a response to social interpretations which prevent cystics and their families from learning the therapy techniques and perceiving and enjoying its effects, with central emphasis on the notion that social interpretations are improvised in response to real or imagined inexpediences.

In summary, biological factors are surely involved in most cases, but the heart of compliance lies deeper, in the sense of the personal responsibility of each member of the cystic fibrosis network, in their fundamental perspective on the problems, and in the value priorities each establishes while improvising social interpretations in the face of real or presumed forces of social control at each step in the emergence of compliance. It is not primarily factors such as effective communication between health providers and patients or health beliefs in the seriousness of the disease and the efficacy of care that motivate compliance; characteristics of patients, regimes and illnesses do not enable one to predict poor compliance. Gradually, by social interpretations improvised in the face of the forces of social control, the techniques of cystic fibrosis therapy are learned and its effects are perceived and enjoyed. It is during this process that compliance emerges as the central feature of a cystic fibrotic's life; his inevitable non-compliance is equally central and cannot be dismissed.

CONCLUSION

The term "improvisation" conceptualises the emergent nature of compliance with cystic fibrosis therapy better than do the common mechanistic views of compliance. Davis (1963) used this term with reference to polio victims' reactions over a period of time to their disease, its treatment and effects. For

persons afflicted with chronic life-threatening illnesses, this period of time is their life. Mechanistic views with their attempts to predict and to
motivate compliance fail to conceptualise fully these
children's life-long improvisations.

Clearly, compliance with therapy for any chronic
life-threatening illness will be enhanced only by
clearer conceptualisations of its emergent nature. As
medical sociology matures, attempts at such conceptualisation should be encouraged in conjunction with
the mechanistic views.

With clearer conceptualisation, more complete evaluation of medical regimes is possible (Soutter and
Kennedy, 1974). Such an evaluation is attempted in
the following chapter.

5

EVALUATING THE WORTH OF THERAPY

Critics of prophylactic therapy for cystic fibrosis cite the strain its time-consuming nature and intensity generates in the family; there are two hours a day of active physio- and inhalation-therapy. Furthermore, they question the worth of a regime that frequently postpones death from early childhood unawareness until late adolescent awareness. Proponents, however, argue that this price is not as much as one would pay if one neglected treatment or used it intermittently; the slow and relentless decline of a child with racking cough and gasping breath is anything but peaceful. They posit that what is earned from prophylactic therapy is the increasing chance to have children who grow up into adults of normal appearance and activity.

For example, in 1950, more than 80 per cent of the children diagnosed cystic fibrotic died before they reached their first birthday; today, with early diagnosis and optimal treatment, 80 per cent reach their 19th year (Shwachman and Holsclaw, 1969; and Anderson and Goodchild, 1976). Such survival rates are reported from Melbourne, London and throughout the United States (Anderson, 1967; Huang et al., 1970; Warwick and Monson, 1967; Warwick and Poque, 1969; Shwachman et al., 1965; Mikkelsen et al., 1978; and Anderson, 1978). Gurry (1975) quotes data from the

Cleveland Cystic Fibrosis Clinic: a 100 per cent survical up to 12 years of age for all cases diagnosed at birth and given intensive prophlactic therapy.

Critics hold the view that the prognosis for the quality of life in young adult cystics is so poor that it offsets the prognosis for longevity. Anderson and Goodchild (1976), among others, disagree. They cite Shwachman's *et al*. (1974) study of 70 patients over 25 years of age: twenty-eight were married and 6 of the women had children; forty graduated from tertiary institutions; there were 13 who held Masters degrees, one who was a medical doctor, two lawyers, three nurses, a physiotherapist and an engineer. Apart from the fact that 100 per cent of the males were aspermic and 50 per cent of the sample had nasal polyposis, physical complications were impalpable. Proponents of cystic fibrosis therapy argue that these findings give some indication of the quality of life in adulthood which can be achieved.

Finally, critics claim that longevity and quality of life are due to earlier and wider diagnosis of milder variants of the disease; thus doubt cast on the value of intensive treatment is not effaced. Proponents agree that early and wide diagnosis promotes longevity and quality of life; neonatal screening procedures are proposed (Brimblecome and Chamberlain, 1973; Brune *et al*., 1974; Anderson and Goodchild, 1976; and Anderson, 1978). However, they argue that milder variants of cystic fibrosis do not obviate the need for intensive prophylactic treatment but enhance its need in maintaining healthy lives.

As with the evaluation of therapies for many other
chronic life-threatening illnesses, this evaluation of
cystic fibrosis therapy is systematic and precise,
yields measures of longevity and quality of life and
has the widespread support of evaluation research
methodologists (Nutt, 1981; Schulberg et al., 1969;
Gordon and Morse, 1975; Sax, 1972; Rutman, 1977; and
Guttentag and Struening, 1975). Nevertheless, the
results of this evaluation are not conclusive. Not
only are there operationalisation problems in the
measurement of the quality of life but there are
frequently political and economic controversies over
the establishment of cystic fibrosis clinics; some-
times competition for monies and kudos among medical
personnel for their particular child care service is
fierce (Perrow, 1961; Rossi and Wright, 1977;
Mechanic, 1975; McAuliffe, 1979; and Wildavsky, 1977).
Furthermore, by and large neglected in this debate on
the worth of therapy for children growing up with
cystic fibrosis, cancer or muscular dystrophy are the
thoughts of the recipients of the treatment (cf.
Strauss and Glaser, 1975). The purpose of this
chapter is to mitigate partially this neglect.

THE RECIPIENTS OF THERAPY

Initially, I thought that cystics would reply with
unequivocal affirmation to a question of this sort:
"Is your cystic fibrosis therapy worth it?" However,
it appeared that responses were largely a function of
emotional or physical conditions at the time. Further
scrutiny qualified this impression.

The chaos of many situation-specific responses could be interpreted as a continuous and systematic evaluation of the treatment based upon highly calculable faith/hope exchanges but with impromptu assessments. That is, while there are many individualised evaluations of therapy, they may be synthesised into a simplified proposition of exchange theory (Thibaut and Kelley, 1959; Homans, 1958; Blau, 1964; and Emerson, 1976): a person will continue to participate with another person only as long as the inducements he receives are as great as or greater than the contributions he is asked to make, and more favourable alternatives are not open to him. In other words, a person afflicted with cystic fibrosis may continue to favourably value intensive preventative therapy only so long as he perceives that the hope he receives is as great as or greater than the faith he gives within the cystic fibrosis network of relationships, and more favourable alternatives are not perceived to be open to him.

Thus a healthy cystic who receives a high degree of hope from her family evaluates her therapy very favourably. On the other hand, another reportedly healthy cystic finds little value in the intensive preventative therapy regime; he is preparing to transfer from child health services to adult health services. Another case is that of a young girl with cystic fibrosis who has a poor prognosis, is frequently hospitalised and has a persistent cough, yet, she values her therapy highly:

> The best thing about being sick is that
> everybody takes care of you. Mummy and
> daddy visit every day and all sorts of
> people take care of me ... When I get better
> I'm going to be a sister (nurse) or
> something so that I can take care of kids
> like me.

Thus, for a person afflicted with cystic fibrosis, it does not appear to be solely the consequences of the treatment, but the faith/hope exchange in which melieu the treatment occurs that may largely determine their evaluation of prophylactic therapy.

The value of the faith/hope exchange is relative to the significance other members in the cystic fibrosis network have to each cystic. That is, cystics calculate the faith given and hope received not so much in direct terms but in terms of with whom the exchange takes place. Paraphrasing a paediatrician to illustrate:

> I don't think they (the children) realise
> the full value of this treatment. They
> become very complacent. But if they trust
> one of us a great deal they'll do anything
> we ask. But let that person let them down
> and we're lost. We have to start from
> scratch building up a relationship with the
> parents, the kids; encouraging them. It's
> all based on personal relationships - or at
> least 99 per cent of it is ... So if one
> particular nurse, let's say, is well liked,
> she makes certain to say "hello". We all
> know how important personal relationships
> are here in keeping up with treatment.

CONCLUSION

In conclusion, for children growing up with a life-threatening illness the evaluation of therapy is a continually emerging process of their very existence. The actual or potential consequences are not the sole criteria they use in evaluating the worth of therapy; rather, the value of the net effects of therapy seems to be mediated through an exchange of symbols - meanings and definitions. The relevant symbols are faith and hope which they exchange with other members of the therapeutic network throughout the situation-specific emotional and physical conditions experienced while growing up with the disease; the value of faith and hope is relative to the significance other members have to the individual child.

Vernon (1978) offers a symbolic interaction paradigm which conceptualises this evaluation process. He argues that an individual's social behaviour is in response to symbols relative to audiences and situations; he capitalises this paradigm: ISAS. Cystic fibrotics' evaluation of therapy may be viewed as a form of social behaviour. Viewed in this way, the evaluation of intensive prophylactic therapy is in response to the exchange of faith and hope, relative to other members in the cystic fibrosis network and to the emotional and physical situations that comprise the life of a person growing up with cystic fibrosis.

Thus, the final evaluation of intensive medical treatment of cystic fibrosis, and perhaps treatment of any other chronic illness or handicap is not complete solely by assessing its medical and social consequences or potential consequences; questioning the recipients as well as the dispensors of therapy is required. As patient participation in medical care increases (Friedman and Di Matteo, 1979; Hayes-Bautis, 1976; and Levine and Kozloff, 1978) this type of evaluation research needs to be encouraged in conjunction with the more traditional forms of assessment.

6

A POSTSCRIPT: FIELD RESEARCH IN MEDICAL SOCIOLOGY

This research experience has convinced me that if we are to make a major advance in our understanding of the ill, in conjunction with survey and experimental designs we must undertake field research whereby we look, listen and feel with these people. To do this is an ambitious undertaking and one not without problems:

1. presenting representative and reliable data and testable theory (cf. Cuff and Payne, 1979) and

2. coping with feelings of personal inefficacy.

Nevertheless, it is a valuable undertaking.

Methodologically, field research may not be the sole basis upon which to build medical sociology but certainly it is a necessity without which medical sociologists would be myopic. Feelings of personal inefficacy do not preclude the fact that the results of field research may be useful to the ill. Field research is a tool for sociological understanding; the utility of such understanding depends not only on tools but also upon craftsmanship (Polsky, 1971; and Glaser and Strauss, 1967).

FIELD RESEARCH

Field research is inductive. For this reason, in medical sociology it is most prominent in debunking existing sociological understanding rather than for theory construction. A common example of this prominence is with Parsons' (1951 and 1975) "sick role" formulation (e.g. Kosa and Robertson, 1969; and Berkanovic, 1972). However, field research is not the only method used to repudiate, among other factors, the "mediococentric" nature of Parsons' (1951 and 1975) framework; researchers using survey and experimental designs commonly conclude that Parsons over-estimated the therapeutic impact of the physician and the medical institution (cf. Gallagher, 1976; Wilson and Bloom, 1972; Freidson, 1965; and Levine and Kozloff, 1978). These criticisms of the sick role are pertinent to chronic conditions, particularly to life-threatening ones with which children grow up and physical and mental impairments where medical as well as familial and para-familial personnel are involved in therapy (Kassebaum and Bauman, 1965; Cogswell and Weir, 1964; Petroni, 1969; Cockerham, 1978; Bynder and New, 1976; Gordon, 1966; Callahan *et al.*, 1966; Levine and Kozloff, 1978; and Greenley, 1972).

Medical field research is, however, not without a strong theory-constructing impulse. This impulse, although frequently not articulated, is most notable for providing an understanding of the chronically ill and the physically and mentally handicapped.

This theoretical impulse may be best called a situational approach and it provides a similar theoretical perspective to that which Sansom (1980) used in his study of Aboriginal fringe dwellers in Darwin. Within this perspective, human behaviour is viewed as a reasoned form of social behaviour. In order to understand this behaviour one must understand:

1. the logic ascribed to it by the actors;

2. that the actors base their logic upon what they perceive to be real rather than upon external reality *per se;* and

3. that these perceptions of reality are negotiated - created, maintained and transformed - through social interaction (Berger and Luckman, 1967; Schutz, 1970; Natanson, 1974; Giddens, 1976; and Strauss *et al.,* 1964).

Thus, the chronically ill, physically handicapped and mentally impaired do not react directly to their economic, social, psychological and physical conditions. Rather, they continuously ascribe a logic to their behaviour based upon their negotiated perceptions of these conditions. The negotiations take place implicitly within their network of relationships. The logic may be kaleidoscopic but, for the moment at least, it is compelling to the ill person. Roth's (1963) tuberculosis patients with their "bench marks" and their "timetable conflicts" with physicians, Davis' (1963) polio victims with their "improvisations" as they "pass through crisis" and Edgerton's (1967) mentally retarded attempting to "pass" and the "benevolent conspiracy" that transpires are classic studies within medical sociology that capture this logic.

Capturing this logic is the purpose of field research. By knowing their logic, we obtain a sociological understanding of what it is like to have tuberculosis or polio or to be mentally retarded.

Through capturing the logic of the faith for hope exchange at least a partial understanding of what it is like to grow up with a life-threatening illness may have been achieved.

*   *   *   *   *   *   *   *   *   *

REFERENCES

Allan, J. L., R. R. Townley and P. D. Phelan

    1974   "Family response to cystic fibrosis."
             Australian Paediatric Journal 10:136-146

Anderson, C. M.

    1967   "Long term study of patients with cystic
             fibrosis." *Modern Problems of Paediatrics*
             10:344-349

Anderson, C. M. and M. C. Goodchild

    1976   *Cystic Fibrosis: Manual of Diagnosis and
             Management.* Oxford: Blackwell

Anderson, R. W.

    1978   "Cystic fibrosis." Pp. 344-348 in R. M.
             Goldenson, J. R. Dunham and C. S. Dunham
             (eds), *Disability and Rehabilitation
             Handbook.* New York: McGraw-Hill.

Baker, L.

    1978   *You and Leukaemia: A Day at a Time.*
             Philadelphia: W. B. Saunders.

Batten, J.

    1966   "C. F. and the teenager." *Cystic Fibrosis
             News.* (June).

Beall, R. J.

    1981   "Recent publicity concerning potential
              Heterozygote test." Memorandum of the
              Cystic Fibrosis Foundation, Rockville,
              Maryland (January 2):1-4.

Becker, H. S.

    1953   "Becoming a marihuana user." *The American
              Journal of Sociology* LIX (November):235-242.

Becker, M. H. and L. A. Maiman

    1975   Sociobehavioral determinants of compliance
              with health and medical care recommenda-
              tions." *Medical Care* XIII:10-24.

    1980   "Strategies for enhancing patient
              compliance." *Journal of Community Health*,
              6:113-135.

Berger, P. L.

    1969   *The Sacred Canopy.* Garden City: Anchor.

Berger, P. L. and H. Kellner

    1970   "Marriage and the construction of reality:
              An exercise in the microsociology of
              knowledge." Pp. 50-72 in H. P. Dreitzel
              (ed.) *Recent Sociology No. 2.* New York:
              Macmillan.

Berger, P. L. and T. Luckman

    1967   *The Social Construction of Reality.* Garden
              City: Anchor.

Berkanovic, E.

   1972   "Lay conceptions of the sick role." *Social
           Forces* 51:53-63.

Beveridge, J. and P. Lykke

   1973   "Psychological stress due to cystic
           fibrosis." A paper presented at the
           meetings of The Australian Paediatric
           Association, Canberra, A.C.T. (April).

Blau, P. M.

   1964   *Exchange and Power in Social Life.* New
           York: Wiley.

Breslow, J. L., J. McPherson, J. Epstein

   1981   "Distinguishing homozygous and heterozygous
           cystic fibrosis fibroblasts from normal
           cells by difference in sodium transport."
           New England Journal of Medicine 304, 1:1-5.

Brimblecombe, F. S. W. and J. Chamberlain

   1973   Screening for cystic fibrosis." *Lancet*
           1428-1431.

Brune, W. T., T. R. Cornell, J. A. Lacey and W. E.
Whisler

   1974   "A one year screening study for cystic
           fibrosis with the B.M.C. test in sixteen
           thousand newborn infants." *1975 Cystic
           Fibrosis Club Abstract* 13, 3 (September).

Burton, L.

   1975   *The Family Life of Sick Children.* London:
           Routledge and Kegan Paul.

Bury, M.

    1982   "Chronic illness as biographical
                 disruption." *Sociology of Health and
                 Illness*, 4,2:167-182.

Bynder, H. and P. K. New

    1976   "Time for a change: From micro- to
                 macro-sociological concepts in disability
                 research." *Journal of Health and Social
                 Behaviour* 17:45-52.

Callahan, E. M., S. Carroll, S. P. Revier, E. Gilhooly
and D. Dunn

    1966   "The 'sick role' in chronic illness: Some
                 reactions." *Journal of Chronic Diseases*
                 19:883-897.

Cassell, E. J.

    1978   *The Healer's Art*. Middlesex: Penguin.

Charney, E.

    1972   "Patient-doctor communication: Implications
                 for clinician." *Paediatric Clinics of North
                 America*, 19:263-279.

Cockerham, W. C.

    1978   *Medical Sociology*. Englewood Cliffs:
                 Prentice-Hall.

Cogswell, B. E. and D. D. Weir

    1964   "A role in process: The development of
                 medical professionals' role in long term
                 care of chronically diseased patients."
                 Journal of Health and Social Behaviour
                 5:95-103.

Cook, C. D., P. J. Hellicsen, L. Kulczycki, H. Barrie,
L. Friedlanders, S. Agathon, G. B. C. Harris and
H. Schwachman

    1959   "Lung volumes and mechanics of respiration
               in 64 patients with cystic fibrosis of the
               pancreas." *Paediatrics* 24:181.

Cuff, E. C. and G. C. F. Payne (eds)

    1979   *Perspectives in Sociology.* London: George
               Allen and Unwin.

Cummings, S. T., H. C. Bayley and H. E. Rie

    1966   "Effects of the child's deficiency on the
               mother: A study of mothers of mentally
               retarded, chronically ill and neurotic
               children." *American Journal of
               Orthopsychiatry* 36:595-608.

Danks, D. M., J. Allan and C. M. Anderson

    1965   "A genetic study of fibrocystic disease
               of the pancreas." *Annals of Human Genetics*
               28:323-356.

Davis, F.

    1960   "Uncertainty in medical prognosis-clinical
               and functional" *American Journal of
               Sociology* 66:41-47.

    1961   "Deviance disavowal: The management of
               strained interaction by the visiby handi-
               capped." *Social Problems* 9:121-132.

    1963   *Passage Through Crisis: Polio Victims and
               Their Families.* Indianapolis:
               Bobbs-Merrill.

Davis, M.

    1973   *Living with Multiple Sclerosis.*
                Springfield: Charles C. Thomas.

Davis, M. I.

    1968   "Physiological, psychological and
                demographic factors in patient compliance
                with doctors' orders." *Medical Care*
                XI:115-122.

Davis, M. S. and R. L. Eichhorn

    1963   "Compliance with medical care regimens:
                A panel study." *Journal of Health and*
                Human Behavior 4:240-249.

De Jong, W.

    1980   "The stigma of obesity: The consequences
                of naive assumptions concerning the cause
                of physical deviance." *Journal of Health*
                and Social Behavior 21 (March):75-87.

Dingwall, R.

    1976   *Aspects of Illness.* London: Martin
                Robertson.

Doyle, B.

    1959   "Physical therapy in the treatment of
                cystic fibrosis." *Physical Therapy Review*
                39:24-27.

Edgerton, R. B.

    1967   *The Cloak of Competence.* Berkeley:
                University of California Press.

Edwards, C.

1966   "Cystic fibrosis and the medical social
        worker," *Cystic Fibrosis News* (November).

Emerson, R. M.

1976   "Social exchange theory." Pp.335-362 in
        A. Inkeles, J. Coleman and N. Smelser (eds),
        Annual Review of Sociology 2. Palo Alto:
        Annual Reviews.

Fox, R.

1976   "Advanced medical technology - Social and
        ethical implications." Pp.231-268 in A.
        Inkeles, J. Coleman and N. Smelser (eds).
        Annual Review of Sociology 2. Palo Alto:
        Annual Reviews.

Frank III, A. W.

1979   "Reality construction in interaction."
        Pp.167-191 in A. Inkeles, J. Coleman and
        R. H. Turner (eds), *Annual Review of
        Sociology*, 5. Palo Alto: Annual Reviews.

Freidson, E.

1965   Disability and social deviance." Pp.71-99
        in M. B. Sussman (ed), *Sociology and
        Rehabilitation*. Washington, D.C.: American
        Sociological Association.

Friedman, H. S. and M. R. DiMatteo

1979   "Health care as an interpersonal process."
        The Journal of Social Issues 35,1:1-11.

Frydman, M. I.

    1980   "Social class-related correlates of parents'
            knowledge of cystic fibrosis." A paper
            presented at the annual meetings of the
            Sociological Association of Australia and
            New Zealand, Hobart, Tasmania (August).

Gallagher, E. B.

    1976   "Lines of reconstruction and extension in
            the Parsonian sociology of illness."
            Social Science and Medicine 10:207-218.

Giddens, A.

    1976   *New Rules of the Sociological Method.*
            London: Hutchinson.

Glaser, B. G. and A. L. Strauss

    1965   *Awareness of Dying.* Chicago: Aldine.

    1967   *The Discovery of Grounded Theory.* Chicago:
            Aldine.

    1968   *Time for Dying.* Chicago: Aldine.

Goffman, E.

    1959   *The Presentation of Self in Everyday Life.*
            Garden City: Anchor.

    1961   *Encounters: Two Studies in the Sociology
            of Interaction.* Indianapolis:
            Bobbs-Merrill.

    1963   *Stigma: Notes on the Management of Spoiled
            Identity.* Englewood Cliffs: Prentice-Hall.

    1967   *Interaction Ritual.* Garden City:
            Doubleday.

Gordon, G.

1966   *Role Theory and Illness: A Sociological
        Perspective*. New Haven: College
        University.

Gordon, G. and E. V. Morse

1975   "Evaluation research".   Pp.339-361 in
        A. Inkeles, J. Coleman and N. Smelser (eds),
        Annual Review of Sociology 1.   Palo Alto:
        Annual Reviews.

Greenley, J. R.

1972   "The psychiatric patient's family and length
        of hospitalisation." *Journal of Health
        and Social Behavior* 13:25-37.

Gurry, D. L.

1975   "Management of children with cystic
        fibrosis." *Australian Paediatric Journal*
        11:89-90.

Gussow, Z. and G. S. Tracy

1968   "Status, ideology, and adaption to
        stigmatized illness: A study of leprosy."
        Human Organisation 27:316-325.

Guttentag, M. and E. L. Struening (eds)

1975   *Handbook of Evaluation Research*, Vols 1
        and 2. London: Sage.

Hayes-Bautista, D. E.

1976   "Modifying the treatment: Patient
        compliance, patient control and medical
        care." *Social Science and Medicine*
        10:233-238.

Holsclaw, D. W.

1970   "Common pulmonary complications of cystic
        fibrosis." *Clinical Paediatrician*
        9:346-335.

Homans, C. G.

1978   "Social behavior as exchange." *American
        Journal of Sociology* 62:597-606.

Huang, N. (ed)

1972   *Guide to Drug Therapy in Treatment of Cystic
        Fibrosis.* Atlanta: Cystic Fibrosis
        Foundation.

Huang, N. N., C. N. Macri, J. Girone and A. Sproul

1970   "Survival of patients with cystic fibrosis."
        American Journal of Disabled Children
        120:289-295.

Kassebaum, G. G. and B. O. Bauman

1965   "Dimensions of the sick role in chronic
        illness." *Journal of Health and Social
        Behavior* 6:16-27.

Kosa, J. and L. S. Robertson

1969   "The social aspects of health and illness."
        Pp.35-68 in J. Kosa, A. Antonovsky and
        K. Zola (eds), *Poverty and Health.*
        Cambridge:
        Harvard University.

Kubler-Ross, E.

1978   *On Death and Dying.* London: Tavistock.

Kulczycki, L. L.

1970   "Adequate home care for patients with cystic
        fibrosis." *Clinical Proceedings of the
        Children's Hospital*, Washington, D.C.
        25:320-324.

Kulczycki, L. L., M. Robinson and C. Berg

1969   "Somatic and psychological factors relative
        to management of patients with CF."
        *Clinical Proceedings of the Children's
        Hospital*, Washington, D.C. 25:320-324.

Kulczycki, L. L. and H. Shwachman

1958   "Studies in cystic fibrosis of the pancreas:
        Occurrence of rectal prolapse." *New
        England Journal of Medicine* 259:409-412.

Lawler, R. H., W. Nakielny and N. Wright

1966   "Psychological implications of cystic
        fibrosis." *Canadian Medical Association
        Journal* (May) 94:1043-1046.

Levine, S. and M. A. Kozloff

1978   "The sick role: Assessment and overview."
        Pp.317-343 in R. H. Turner, J. Coleman and
        R. C. Fox (eds). *Annual Review of
        Sociology* 4. Palo Alto: Annual Reviews.

McAuliffe, W. E.

1979   "Measuring the quality of medical care:
        Process versus outcome." *Milbank Memorial
        Fund Quarterly* 57:118-152.

McCollum, A. T.

    1971   "Cystic fibrosis: Economic impact upon
               the family." *American Journal of Public
               Health* 61:1335-1340.

McCollum, A. T., and L. E. Gibson

    1970   "Family adaptation to the child with cystic
               fibrosis." *Paediatrics* 77:571-578.

McCrae, W. M., A. M. Cull, L. Burton and J. Dodge

    1973   "Cystic fibrosis: Parents' response to
               the genetic basis of the disease." *Lancet*,
               2:141-143.

McKercher, P. L. and T. D. Rucker

    1977   "Patient knowledge and compliance with
               medication instruction." *Journal of the
               American Pharmaceutical Association*
               17:282-286.

Marston, M.

    1970   "Compliance with medical regimens: A review
               of the literature." *Nursing Research*
               19:312-323.

Matthews, L. W., B. C. Hilman and P. Nathan

    1969   *Vocational and Life Adjustment
               Problems of Young Adults with Cystic
               Fibrosis.* Atlanta: Cystic Fibrosis
               Foundation.

Mearns, M. B.

    1970   "Aerosol therapy in cystic fibrosis."
               Archives of Diseases of Childhood 45:605-607

Mechanic, D.

1975   "The comparative study of health care
        delivery systems." Pp. 43-65 in A. Inkeles,
        J. Coleman and N. Smelser (eds) *Annual
        Review of Sociology* 1. Palo Alto: Annual
        Reviews.

Meyerowitz, J. H. and H. B. Kaplan

1967   "Family response to stress: The case of
        cystic fibrosis." *Social Science and
        Medicine* 1:249.

Mikkelsen, C., E. Waechter and M. Crittenden

1978   "Cystic fibrosis: A family challenge."
        Children Today 7, 4 (July-August):22-26.

Mitchell, J. H.

1974   Compliance with medical regimens: An
        annotated bibliography." *Health Education
        Monograph* 2.

Natanson, M.

1974   *Phenomenology, Role and Reason.*
        Springfield: Thomas.

Nutt, P. C.

1981   *Evaluation Concepts and Methods: Shaping
        Policy for the Health Administrator.*
        Jamaica, New York: Spectrum.

Parker, M. and D. Mauger

1979   *Children with Cancer: A Handbook for
        Families and Helpers.* Auckland: Cassell.

Parsons, T.

    1951   *The Social System*. Glencoe: Free Press.

    1975   "The sick role and the role of the physician reconsidered." *Milbank Memorial Fund Quarterly* 53:257-278.

Perrow, C.

    1961   "The Analysis of goals in complex organisation." *American Sociological Review* 26:854-866.

Petroni, F. A.

    1969   "Significant others and illness behaviour: A much neglected sick role contingency." *Sociological Quarterly* 10:32-41.

Pines, M.

    1978   "Tests to forestall hereditary disease." *New York Times Weekly Review* (May 14):8.

Pinkerton, P.

    1969   "Managing the psychological aspects of CF." *Arizona Medicine* 26:348-351.

Polsky, N.

    1971   *Hustlers, Beats and Others*. Ringwood, Victoria: Penguin.

Pryor, J. A., B. A. Webber, M. E. Hodson and J. C. Batten

    1979   Evaluation of the forced expiration techniques as an adjunct to postural drainage in treatment of cystic fibrosis." *British Medical Journal* (18 August), 2 (6187): 417-418.

Rossi, P. H. and S. R. Wright

    1977   "Evaluation research: An assessment of
             theory, practice and politics." *Evaluation*
             Quarterly (February);5-52.

Roth, J. A.

    1963   *Timetables*. Indianapolis: Bobbs-Merrill.

Rutman, L. (ed)

    1977   *Evaluation Research Methods: A Basic Guide*.
             London: Sage.

Sackett, D. L. and R. B. Haynes (eds)

    1976   *Compliance with Therapeutic Regimens*.
             Baltimore: John Hopkins University Press.

Sansom, B.

    1980   *The Camp at Wallaby Cross*. Canberra:
             Australian Institute of Aboriginal Studies.

Sax, S.

    1972   *Medical Care in the Melting Pot: An
             Australian Review*. Sydney: Angus and
             Robertson.

Schulberg, H. C., A. Sheldon and F. Baker

    1969   *Program Evaluation in the Health Field*.
             New York: Behavioral Publications.

Schutz, A.

    1970   *On Phenomenology and Social Relations*.
             Chicago: Chicago University.

Shwachman, H. and D. S. Holsclaw

  1969   "Complications of cystic fibrosis." *New England Journal of Medicine* 281:500-501

Shwachman, H., M. Kowalski and K. T. Khaw

  1974   "70 patients with cystic fibrosis over 25 years of age - a new outlook." *Cystic Fibrosis Club Abstract* 13, 3.

Shwachman, H., L. L. Kulczycki and K. T. Khaw

  1965   "Studies in cystic fibrosis: Report on sixty-five patients over 17 years of age." *Paediatrics* 36:689-699.

Soutter, B. R. and M. C. Kennedy

  1974   "Patient compliance assessment in drug trials: Usage and methods." *Australia, New Zealand Journal of Medicine* 4:360-364.

Spock, A., H. M. Heick, H. Cress and W. S. Logan

  1967   "Abnormal serum factor in patients with cystic fibrosis of the pancreas." *Paediatric Research* 1:173-177.

Spock, A. and D. J. Stedman

  1966   "Psychological characteristics of children with cystic fibrosis." *North Carolina Medical Journal* (September):426-428.

Stone, G. C.

  1979   "Patient compliance and the role of the expert." *Journal of Social Issues 35,* 1:34-59.

Straus, R.

1957   "The nature and status of medical
        sociology." *American Sociological Review*
        22 (April):200-204.

Strauss, A. L.

1959   *Mirrors and Masks: The Search for Identity.*
        Glencoe: Free Press.

Strauss, A. L. and B. G. Glaser

1975   *Chronic Illness and the Quality of Life.*
        Saint Louis: Mosby.

Strauss, A. L., L. Schatzman, R. Bucher, D. Erlich
and K. Sabshin

1964   *Psychiatric Ideologies and Institutions.*
        Glencoe: Pree Press

Strong, P. M.

1979   *The Ceremonial Order of the Clinic:
        Parents, Doctors and Medical Bureaucracies.*
        London: Routledge and Kegan Paul.

Sudnow, D.

1967   *Passing On: The Social Organization of
        Dying.* Englewood Cliffs: Prentice-Hall.

Sykes, G. M. and D. Matza

1957   "Techniques of neutralization: A theory
        of delinquency." *American Sociological
        Review* 22 (December):664-670.

Tecklin, J. S. and D. S. Holsclaw

    1973   "Cystic fibrosis and the role of the
              physical therapist in its management."
              Physical Therapy 53, 4 (April):186-393.

Teicher, J. D.

    1969   "Psychological aspects of cystic fibrosis
              in children and adolescents." *California
              Medical Journal* 110:371-374.

Thibaut, J. and H. H. Kelley

    1959   *The Social Psychology of Groups.* New York:
              Wiley.

Tropauer, A., M. N. Franz and V. W. Dilgard

    1970   "Psychological aspects of the care of
              children with cystic fibrosis." *American
              Journal of Diseases in Children* 119:424-432

Turk, J.

    1964   "Impact of Cystic Fibrosis on family
              functioning." *Paediatrics* (July):67-71.

Twaddle, A. C.

    1982   "From medical sociology to the sociology
              of health: Some changing concerns in the
              sociological study of sickness and
              treatment." Pp. 323-358 in T. Bottomore,
              S. Nowak and M. Sokolowska (eds.) *Sociology:
              The State of the Art.* London: Sage.

Vernon, G. M.

    1978   *Symbolic Aspects of Interaction.*
              Washington, D.C.: University Press of
              America.

Voysey, M.

    1972   "Impression management by parents with
              disabled children." *Journal of Health and
              Social Behaviour* 13:80-89.

Waddell, H.

    1933   *Peter Abelard*. London: Constable.

Warwick, W. J. and S. Monson

    1967   "Life table studies of mortality." *Modern
              Problems of Paediatrics* 10:353-367.

Warwick, W. J. and R. E. Poque

    1969   "Computer studies in cystic fibrosis."
              P.320 in *Proceedings of the Fifth
              International CF Conference*. Cambridge:
              Cystic Fibrosis Research Trust.

Wildavsky, A.

    1977   "Doing better and feeling worse: The
              political pathology of health policy."
              Daedalus 106 (Winter):105-123.

Wilson, R. N. and S. W. Bloom

    1972   "Patient-practitioner relationships."
              Pp. 315-339 in H. E. Freeman, S. Levine
              and L. G. Reeder (eds) *Handbook of Medical
              Sociology*. Englewood Cliffs:
              Prentice-Hall.

Zola, I. K.

    1966   "Culture and symptoms: An analysis of
              patients' presenting complaints." *American
              Sociological Review* 31:615-630.

ABOUT THE AUTHOR

Charles Waddell, Ph.D. (Utah), is a lecturer in Anthropology and Sociology at the University of Western Australia, Perth. His main research interests are in the sociology of health and illness. He has just completed a study on the length of hospitalisation of Australian Aboriginal children and is currently studying the utilisation of orthodox and unorthodox health services in Western Australia. He shares these interests with his wife, Vivienne, a medical practitioner. They have a two year old son, Gregory.